HOW TO STOP AND REVERSE HEART DISEASE

Understanding Your Heart, Risk Factors, and Solutions

COPYRIGHT

CATALOG

Part 1 ...3

Your Heart ...3

A Vital Engine ...3

Chapter 1 ...4

Learning About the Heart's Structure and Function ...4

Chapter 2 ...14

How Your Heart Works ...14

From the Beat to the Blood Flow ...14

Part 2 ...24

The Threat ...24

Unveiling Heart Disease ...24

Chapter 3 ...25

Heart Disease: What It Is, Why It Happens, and How It Can Get Worse ...25

Chapter 4 ...32

Atherosclerosis and Plaque Buildup ...32

The Silent Killer ...32

Part 3 ...40

Knowing Your Enemy ...40

Risk Factors for Heart Disease ...40

Chapter 5 ...41

Risk Factors You Can't Change ...41

Genetics, Age, and Family History ...41

Chapter 6 ...47

Risk Factors That Can Be Changed ...47

Lifestyle Choices You Can Make ...47

Part 4 ...56

Taking Charge ...56

Strategies for Stopping Heart Disease ...56

Chapter 7 ...57

How to Eat Well for Your Heart ...57

Food as Medicine ...57

A plate of brightly colored fruits and veggies ...58

Chapter 8 64

Move Your Body 64

How Exercise Can Help Your Heart 64

Part 5 ....**71**

Optimizing Your Health **71**

Lifestyle Habits for Prevention **71**

Chapter 9 72

How to Control Your Weight 72

Finding a Healthy Balance 72

Chapter 10 79

Seeing the Enemy 79

Heart Disease Diagnostic Tools 79

Part 6 ....**84**

Beyond Lifestyle **84**

Medical Interventions for Heart Disease **84**

Chapter 11 85

Medicines For Heart Health 85

Learning About Your Choices 85

Chapter 12 90

When Lifestyle Changes Aren't Enough 90

Procedures And Interventions 90

Part 7 ....**95**

Living Well with Heart Disease **95**

A Guide to Long-Term Management **95**

Chapter 13 96

You Will Be Committed To Heart Health For The Rest Of Your Life 96

A promise for life: a heart-healthy future **101**

Chapter 14 103

Keeping Your Physical And Mental Health In Good Shape To Live a
Fulfilling Life 103

Part 1
Your Heart
A Vital Engine

Chapter 1

Learning About the Heart's Structure and Function

The heart, which is inside your chest and works nonstop, is like an engine that keeps everything running. It's amazing how this amazing organ, which is about the size of your fist clenched, constantly pumps blood all over your body, bringing waste and oxygen to every cell. But before we get into the amazing details of how it does this, let's take a look at the heart's complicated structure and the interesting physiology that controls its beat.

Where it is and how it is protected: The Heart's Home

The heart is located in the mediastinum, a hollow spot in the middle of your chest that is between your lungs and leans slightly to the left. Its position in this way makes it easy for it to pump blood to the lungs and the rest of the body.

A sac with two layers around the heart is called the pericardium. The outer layer is called the fibrous pericardium, and it is made up of tough fibers that support the heart and hold it in place against the other organs. The inner layer, called the serous pericardium, makes a fluid that keeps the heart moving smoothly inside the chest cavity when it contracts. This lubrication keeps the heart muscle from getting worn down by rubbing.

There are four rooms in Chambers of the Heart:

Think of the heart as a four-story house, with each room being responsible for a different part of the blood flow. Let's look around these rooms:

There are two upper spaces with thin walls that receive blood. These are called the atria (singular: atrium). Two big veins, the superior and inferior vena cava, bring deoxygenated blood back to the heart through the right atrium. Four pulmonary veins bring oxygenated blood back from the lungs to the left heart.

Ventricles (singular: ventricle): These are the two lower chambers with stronger walls that pump blood through the heart. The heart's right ventricle sends blood that is low on oxygen to the lungs so that gases can be exchanged. Through a network of arteries, the heart's largest chamber, the left ventricle, sends oxygenated blood to every part of the body.

There are one-way valves between the atria and ventricles that make sure blood moves in the right direction. If there is blood flow between the left atrium and ventricle and the right atrium and ventricle, the mitral valve controls it. The tricuspid valve protects the space between the two.

There are a lot of muscles in Walls of the Heart.

The heart has walls made of muscle called the myocardium. These walls are made up of cardiac muscle, a special kind of muscle tissue. You can choose to contract or relax skeletal muscle, but not heart muscle. heart muscle contracts in a rhythmic and constant way without your conscious effort.

This special tissue makes it possible for the heart to beat nonstop, day and night, for the rest of your life.

The myocardium is made up of three layers:

Epicardium: This is the heart's outermost layer. It protects it and joins it to the pericardium.

Myocardium: The cardiac muscle fibers that make the heart pump are in this layer, which is the largest and most important part.

It is the deepest layer of the heart that lines the chambers and valves and makes sure that blood flows smoothly.

The electrical conduction system keeps the heart's rhythm.

Your heart beats in a steady pace that isn't random; it's carefully planned by the electrical conduction system. This specific group of tissues in the heart muscle sends and receives electrical signals that tell the different chambers to contract together.

The electrical impulse is started by the sinoatrial node (SA node), which is also called the pacemaker and is found in the right ventricle. After this energy goes through the atria, it makes them contract, which sends blood to the ventricles. The impulse then goes through the atrioventricular node (AV node), which is a path between the atria and ventricles. The AV node controls the flow of electrical signals in the heart. It delays the signal a little so that the atria can finish contracting before starting the tightening of the ventricles. Lastly, the impulse goes through Purkinje fibers, which are specialized muscle bundles that make sure the muscular walls of the ventricles contract at the same time. This pumps blood out of the heart.

There is only one way to use the Blood Flow Highway

Now that we know how the heart is put together, let's follow the blood as it moves through its chambers:

Blood Return Without Oxygen: Blood that has been carrying oxygen to your body's tissues then leaves them and enters the heart through two big veins, the superior and inferior vena cava.

Right Atrium to Right Ventricle: When the right atrium gets smaller, it squeezes the tricuspid valve, which forces blood into the right ventricle.

Gas Exchange from the Right Ventricle to the Lungs: When the right ventricle contracts, it pushes deoxygenated blood through the pulmonic valve and into the pulmonary artery. The pulmonary artery then splits into two branches, each bringing blood to a lung. Fresh oxygen is taken in by the lungs and carbon dioxide is taken out of the blood.

Oxygenated Blood Return: Four pulmonary veins bring oxygenated blood back to the heart, where it enters the left ventricle.

To get from the left atrium to the left ventricle, the left atrium closes and forces oxygenated blood through the mitral valve and into the heart's strongest chamber, the left ventricle.

Left Ventricle to Body: The left ventricle contracts strongly, pushing oxygenated blood through the aortic valve and into the aorta, the body's biggest artery. A network of arteries breaks off from the aorta and brings oxygen and food to every cell in your body.

The Cycle Continues: The body's deoxygenated blood then flows back to the right heart, where the cycle starts all over again.

There are many valves and sounds that make up the heartbeat.

The sounds we connect with a heartbeat come from the heart chambers contracting in a rhythmic way and the valves opening and closing. Two different sounds, which are often called "lub-dub," can be heard with every heartbeat:

Lub: This is the sound that the tricuspid and mitral valves make when they close and the ventricles get smaller. It is louder and lower in pitch.

Dub: This sound is sharper and higher pitched because the pulmonic and aortic valves are closing. This happens when the ventricles rest and blood flow slows down for a moment.

It is possible to hear these sounds with a stethoscope, a medical tool that lets doctors listen to the heart and find any problems with its beat or function.

A closer look at the pumping action in the heart's cycle

The cardiac cycle is made up of the regulated contractions and relaxations of the heart chambers and the opening and closing of valves. This cycle can be broken down even further into two parts:

This is the phase of rest, and the ventricles are full of blood. When the semilunar valves (pulmonic and aorta) close, blood flows into the ventricles through the atria. At the same time, the atrioventricular valves (tricuspid and mitral) are open.

This is the moment of contraction when the ventricles push blood out of the heart. When the ventricles squeeze, they push the blood toward the arteries. This opens the semilunar valves and closes the atrioventricular valves.

Heart rate, which is given in beats per minute (bpm), shows how many cardiac strokes your heart makes in one minute. Heart rates that are good can change based on age, fitness level, and activity level.

How the Heart Works: Keeping the Beat Stable

Several things work together to keep the heart rate steady and make sure the body gets enough blood to meet its changing needs:

The nervous system: The autonomic nervous system, which is made up of the sympathetic and parasympathetic nervous systems, is very important for keeping the heart rate in check. The sympathetic nervous system speeds up the heart rate when we are stressed or working hard. On the other hand, the parasympathetic nervous system slows the heart rate when we are at ease.

Hormones: Your heart rate can go up when you're stressed or working out because hormones like adrenaline and epinephrine are released.

Blood Chemistry: The amount of electrolytes in the blood, such as calcium and potassium, can change the heart rate and beat.

In conclusion

The human heart is an amazing organ that is carefully designed and controlled to keep us living. By learning about its structure, how its chambers work together to pump blood, and the electrical signals that set its rhythm, we can better appreciate this tireless engine that keeps us alive. With this basic knowledge, we can learn more about how the heart works in health and illness, which is what we will do in the next few chapters.

Chapter 2

How Your Heart Works

From the Beat to the Blood Flow

Using the anatomy we learned in Chapter 1 as a base, let's look more closely at the amazing mechanics of how your heart works. This chapter will explain how the heart's muscle contractions, the one-way flow of blood, and the electrical signals that control this amazing process all work together.

The Power of Contracture: A Muscular Opus

The myocardium, which is made up of muscle walls in the heart, works hard to keep your heart beating regularly. Heart muscle is automatic, which means it contracts and relaxes on its own, unlike skeletal muscles, which you can control with your mind. Because of this one trait, the heart can beat nonstop, day and night, for the rest of your life.

Blood moves through the vascular system because the four chambers of the heart contract together. More closely, let's look at the order of events:

Filling the Chambers (Diastole): The heart starts out in diastole, a state of relaxation. The ventricles are at their most relaxed during this phase, which lets them fill with blood. The superior and inferior vena cava bring blood back from the body that has lost oxygen to the right atrium. At the same time, the pulmonary veins bring fresh blood from the lungs into the left atrium.

In atrial contraction, both atria squeeze together as diastole comes to a close. This gives blood an extra push into the ventricles. But this atrial squeeze isn't necessary for blood flow; it just makes things work better overall.

When the atrium contracts, the ventricles contract with a lot more force. This is called systole. The ventricles' bigger, stronger walls are made for this strong pumping action. The pressure inside the ventricles goes up as they tighten.

To make sure blood flows in the right direction, one-way valves are put between the chambers and open and close at regular intervals. The tricuspid valve on the right side and the mitral valve on the left side close tightly during ventricular contraction. This stops blood from moving back into the atria. The aortic valve on the left ventricle and the pulmonic valve on the right ventricle both open at the same time, letting blood leave the heart.

Blood Ejection: When the ventricles contract strongly and the right valves open, blood is pushed out into the pulmonary artery, which brings deoxygenated blood to the lungs, and the aorta, which brings oxygenated blood to the rest of the body.

Relaxation and Repeat: The ventricles start to relax as they hit their strongest point of contraction. When the pressure inside the ventricles drops, the pulmonic and aorta valves close. This stops blood from going back into the ventricles. The next phase is diastole, which is the filling process.

The electric impulse: a baton for a conductor

The heart muscle's planned and rhythmic contractions don't happen by chance. A special system for conducting electricity inside the heart carefully coordinates them. This method works like a conductor's baton, making sure that each chamber contracts at the right time and in the right order. This makes the pumping action work well.

The most important parts of this device for conducting electricity are

Sinoatrial Node (SA Node): The SA node, which is in the right atrium, starts the electrical surge. It is often called the heart's natural pacemaker. Because of this urge, the heart muscle knows it needs to contract.

There is an AV node, which is located between the atria and ventricles and serves as a relay point. It gets the electrical input from the SA node and slightly slows it down. Because of this delay, the atria have time to finish contracting and push blood into the ventricles before the ventricles contract and pump blood out.

Purkinje Fibers: These are special muscle fibers that send the electrical signal to the muscle walls of the ventricles. This makes sure that the muscles contract in sync and strongly.

The SA node sends out an electrical signal that moves along this path and causes contractions in a certain order:

The electrical surge starts at the SA node.

The impulse moves through the atria, making all of them shrink at the same time.

When the urge gets to the AV node, it takes a little longer to arrive.

The delayed impulse moves through the Purkinje fibers, making the ventricles contract in an organized way. This makes sure that blood flows smoothly.

A More In-Depth Look at Blood Flow in the Heart

The cardiac cycle is made up of the regulated contractions and relaxations of the heart chambers and the opening and closing of valves. As we talked about in Chapter 1, this cycle can be broken down even further into two separate stages:

When the heart is in diastole (the filling phase), the ventricles rest and the atria squeeze to push blood into the ventricles. At this point, the atrioventricular valves (mitral and tricuspid) are open, letting blood flow from the atria to the ventricles. The semilunar valves (aortic and pulmonic) are closed.

Systole, or "Pumping Phase," is when the heart pumps blood out of the body. The ventricles squeeze hard, pushing blood toward the arteries. When the pressure goes up, the aorta and pulmonic semilunar valves open and the atrioventricular valves close. This stops blood from flowing back into the atria. The ventricles then push blood into the pulmonary artery (which is deoxygenated blood) and the aorta (which is oxygenated blood).

Hearing the beat of life through heart sounds

The sounds we connect with a heartbeat come from the heart chambers contracting in a rhythmic way and the valves opening and closing. It is possible to hear these sounds with a stethoscope, a medical tool that lets doctors listen to the heart and find any problems with its beat or function.

Heart sounds come in two main types:

Lub: This is the louder, lower-pitched sound that the ventricles make when the tricuspid and mitral valves close at the start of systole.

When the pulmonic and aortic valves close at the end of systole, as the ventricles rest, this sound is made. It is sharper and higher in pitch.

A doctor or nurse can tell how healthy and well the heart is working by listening to these sounds and how often they happen.

Things That Affect Heart Rate: Meeting the Needs

Heart rate, which is given in beats per minute (bpm), shows how many cardiac strokes your heart makes in one minute. There are a few things that can change a good heart rate:

Age: A child's heart rate is usually faster than an adult's, and it slows down over time.

Level of Fitness: A heart that is in good shape works better and can pump more blood with fewer beats. This is why the heart rates of athletes often are lower when they are at rest.

Level of Activity: When you're active, your body needs more air and nutrients, so your heart beats faster to meet these needs.

Moods: Anxiety, stress, and joy can all make your heart beat faster.

Body Temperature: If your body temperature is high, your heart rate may be faster.

Medicines: Some medicines can change the heart rate.

The Wonderful Things About Heart Regulation: Keeping Your Balance

Several things work together to keep the heart rate steady and make sure the body gets enough blood to meet its changing needs:

The Nervous System: The autonomic nervous system, which is made up of the sympathetic and parasympathetic nervous systems, is very important. The sympathetic nervous system speeds up the heart rate when we are stressed or working hard. On the other hand, the parasympathetic nervous system slows the heart rate when we are at ease.

Hormones: Your heart rate can go up when you're stressed or working out because hormones like adrenaline and epinephrine are released.

Blood Chemistry: The amount of electrolytes in the blood, such as calcium and potassium, can change the heart rate and beat.

By understanding these control systems, we can realize how amazing it is that the body can fine-tune heart function to meet different needs.

In conclusion

The heart is an amazing piece of tech that was carefully made to pump blood around the body quickly and efficiently. This chapter looked at how electrical impulses, muscle contractions, and the one-way flow of blood all work together to make this important process happen. Knowing how your heart beats and how blood flows through it helps you understand its amazing role in health and illness, which is what we will talk about in the next few chapters.

Part 2

The Threat

Unveiling Heart Disease

Chapter 3

Heart Disease: What It Is, Why It Happens, and How It Can Get Worse

Heart disease, which is a broad term for many diseases that affect the heart, is still the main reason people die around the world. In this chapter, we'll talk about the different kinds of heart disease, their underlying reasons, and the problems that might happen.

Heart disease has many different types. This term shows them all.

Heart disease is not a single thing; it's a general term for a number of illnesses that make it hard for the heart to work properly. Most people have one of these types:

Coronary Artery Disease (CAD) is the type of heart disease that most people have. It happens when plaque, a buildup of fat, forms in the coronary arteries, which carry blood to the heart muscle. This buildup makes the arteries narrow, which lowers blood flow and could cause chest pain or a heart attack.

Heart arrhythmias are problems with the heart's rhythm that can show up as a fast heartbeat (tachycardia), a slow heartbeat (bradycardia), or heartbeats that don't go in a straight line (fibrillation). Depending on the type and intensity, arrhythmias can be harmless or even life-threatening.

Heart failure happens when the heart gets weak and can't pump blood around the body as well as it should. Heart disease, high blood pressure, or damage to the heart muscle are some of the things that can cause it.

Heart Valve Disease: The heart valves keep blood flowing in only one way inside the heart. If these valves get narrowed (stenosis), leaky (regurgitation), or don't work right in some other way, it can affect how blood flows and how the heart works.

Birth Defects of the Heart: These are problems with the heart or important blood vessels that were there at birth. Some defects are small and don't show any signs, but others can be life-threatening and need medical help.

Pericardial Disease: This is when the pericardium, the sac-like tissue that surrounds the heart, gets inflamed or infected. It can make your chest hurt and stop your heart from working right.

Finding the Bad Guys: Heart Disease Risk Factors

Some things that put us at risk for heart disease, like age and family history, we can't change. But a lot of other things we can change about our lifestyle. Here's a better look at the main people to blame:

Unhealthy Diet: Eating a lot of cholesterol, added sugar, saturated and trans fats, and added sugar can make plaque build up in your arteries and raise your chance of coronary artery disease.

Inactivity: Not moving around much makes the heart muscle weaker and raises the risk of becoming overweight, which is another thing that can lead to heart disease.

Smoking: Smoking hurts the walls of blood vessels and raises the chance of blood clots, both of which make coronary artery disease more likely.

Extra Weight and Obesity: Being overweight or obese puts stress on the heart and raises the risk of other health problems, such as high blood pressure and diabetes, which raises the risk of heart disease even more.

High Blood Pressure: When blood pressure is high for a long time, it makes the heart work harder to pump blood, which makes the heart get bigger and weaker over time.

Diabetes: Nerves and blood vessels all over the body, including those that feed the heart, can be hurt by diabetes. Heart disease is much more likely to happen if you have diabetes that you can't control.

High cholesterol: Too much LDL ("bad") cholesterol makes plaque build up in the arteries, while too little HDL ("good") cholesterol helps get rid of LDL cholesterol.

A Chain of Events: Heart Disease Complications That Could Happen

Heart disease can cause many problems, some of which can be life-threatening, if it is not addressed. Here are some possible outcomes:

- A heart attack happens when a blood clot completely stops a coronary artery, cutting off oxygen and food to a part of the heart muscle. Damage to heart muscle during a heart attack can last a long time and cause heart failure.

- A stroke is when a blood clot stops an artery that brings blood to the brain. Heart disease can make blood clots more likely, which means that a stroke could happen.

- We already talked about heart failure, which happens when the heart gets weak and has trouble pumping blood well. It can get worse over time, from mild to serious, which has a big effect on quality of life.

✧ Sudden Cardiac Arrest: This is a dangerous situation in which the heart stops beating quickly and effectively. It can happen at any time, but people with heart problems are more likely to be affected.

✧ Similar to coronary artery disease, peripheral artery disease (PAD) can cause the arteries in the legs and feet to get small. This can happen because of plaque buildup. In the worst cases, this disease can lead to pain, cramps, and even tissue death.

In conclusion

Heart disease is very dangerous because it can come in many forms and can lead to serious problems. But if we know about the different kinds, their underlying causes, and the risk factors that can be changed, we can take steps to avoid them and find them early. The parts that follow will talk about ways to avoid getting heart disease, deal with risk factors, and live a heart-healthy life. We will also talk about the tools used to diagnose and treat different heart problems. If we learn about heart disease and make healthy choices, we can greatly lower our risk of getting it and live longer, better lives.

Chapter 4

Atherosclerosis and Plaque Buildup

The Silent Killer

Coronary artery disease (CAD), which is the most common type of heart disease, is often caused by atherosclerosis, a slowly building up disease in the walls of your vessels. This chapter goes into detail about atherosclerosis and plaque buildup, which can block blood flow to your heart muscle without you knowing it, which could lead to major problems.

Atherosclerosis: A Threat That Comes On Slowly

People with atherosclerosis usually don't notice any signs as the disease gets worse over time. The endothelium, the smooth inner lining of your vessels, acts like a highway for blood flow. This smooth layer gets damaged in atherosclerosis, which sets off a chain of events:

Endothelial Damage: High blood pressure, high cholesterol, smoking, and diabetes are just some of the things that can hurt the endothelial lining of the vessels. This damage makes the surface rough and sticky.

Deposits of fatty acids and inflammation: LDL cholesterol, which is often called "bad" cholesterol, starts to build up in the damaged areas. It starts an inflammatory reaction when these cholesterol particles get stuck in the arterial wall.

Formation of Fatty lines: The trapped LDL cholesterol, white blood cells, and cell debris build up over time, creating fatty lines inside the arterial wall. The first signs of atherosclerosis are these fatty lines.

Plaque Buildup: As the fatty layers get bigger, they can harden and pull in other things, like calcium. Plaque, a thick growth that narrows the artery lumen (inner opening), is made up of this buildup.

Progression and Possible Complications: The buildup of plaque can keep happening, making the artery even narrower and reducing blood flow. Sometimes, the plaque can break, which causes a blood clot to form. If the blood clot forms in a coronary artery, it can block the artery totally, which can cause a heart attack.

If you have atherosclerosis, you might not notice it at first. You might not have any signs until the buildup of plaque cuts off blood flow to the heart muscle so much that you have chest pain (angina) or a heart attack.

Finding the Causes of Risk Factors for Atherosclerosis

Atherosclerosis starts and gets worse because of a number of different causes. While age and family background are risk factors that can't be changed, many others can be changed by making changes to how you live your life:

Unhealthy food: A food high in cholesterol, added sugar, saturated and trans fats, and sodium can make plaque build up faster. For heart health, it's important to eat a lot of fruits, veggies, whole grains, and lean protein.

Physical Inactivity: Heart and blood vessel health are affected by a lack of activity. Blood flow and cholesterol levels stay healthy when you work out regularly.

Smoking: Cigarette smoke hurts the endothelium and raises inflammation, which makes atherosclerosis more likely. One of the most important things you can do to protect your heart health is to stop smoking.

High Blood Pressure: Having high blood pressure all the time makes the heart work harder and can damage the walls of the arteries, making them more likely to get plaque buildup. Keeping blood pressure in a safe range is very important.

Diabetes: Diabetes can hurt blood arteries and make inflammation worse, which speeds up atherosclerosis. Diet, exercise, and medicine are all important ways to control diabetes.

High LDL Cholesterol: Plaque builds up when LDL cholesterol levels are high. On the other hand, HDL cholesterol (the "good" cholesterol) helps clear out the vessels of LDL cholesterol. It's important to work with your doctor to keep your cholesterol numbers in a healthy range.

You can greatly lower your chance of getting atherosclerosis and its possible complications by focusing on these risk factors that you can change.

Finding Atherosclerosis: It's Important to Do It Early

Atherosclerosis often gets worse without anyone noticing, so finding it early is very important. Here are some testing tools that are used to find and rate atherosclerosis:

Exam and Medical History: During the exam, your doctor will talk to you about your medical history, family history, and living habits. A physical check might find signs of high blood pressure or other things that put you at risk.

Blood Tests: Cholesterol, blood sugar, and other signs that can show a higher chance of atherosclerosis can be found in blood tests.

Imaging Tests: Imaging methods such as coronary artery calcium scoring, CT angiography, and echocardiography can show where plaque is accumulating and figure out how small the arteries are.

If atherosclerosis is found early, it can be treated quickly and risk factors can be managed to slow or stop the disease from getting worse.

Fighting atherosclerosis: ways to stop it and take care of it Atherosclerosis can be avoided and is easy to deal with, which is good news. Here are some important plans:

Altering your lifestyle: Eating well, working out regularly, staying at a healthy weight, and dealing with stress are all important ways to stop or slow the development of atherosclerosis.

Medicines: Your doctor may give you medicines to treat atherosclerosis, depending on your risk factors and how bad it is.

Lower LDL cholesterol: Statins are the first thing that should be done to lower LDL cholesterol. You can use other drugs, like ezetimibe or PCSK9 inhibitors, alone or with this one.

Take care of high blood pressure. Drugs like ACE inhibitors, ARBs, diuretics, and beta-blockers can help lower blood pressure and make the heart and vessels less stressed.

Control diabetes: drugs like insulin, metformin, and sulfonylureas can help keep blood sugar levels in check and keep blood vessels from getting damaged.

Stop blood clots: In some cases, aspirin or other blood-thinning drugs may be given to lower the risk of blood clots forming on atherosclerotic plaques.

It is important to remember that medicines work best when used with changes to one's lifestyle.

In conclusion

Atherosclerosis is a threat that nobody sees but can have a big effect on your heart health. You can, however, take charge of your heart health by learning about the risk factors, how plaque builds up, and the different ways to stop it and deal with it. Early detection, along with making healthy lifestyle choices and maybe even taking medicine, can greatly lower your chance of complications like heart attack and stroke. Focus on your heart health and do what you can to keep your arteries clean and your heart healthy.

Part 3

Knowing Your Enemy

Risk Factors for Heart Disease

Chapter 5

Risk Factors You Can't Change

Genetics, Age, and Family History

Many of the things that put you at risk for heart disease can be changed by the choices you make in your daily life. But some things we can't change. This chapter talks about the risk factors for heart disease that you can't change. It also talks about how important early detection and proactive management techniques are, even though these factors can't be changed.

Heart disease risk goes up with age (The March of Time)

Heart disease is definitely more likely to happen as you get older. Several changes in our bodies happen as we age that make us more likely to:

Vessels get stiffer over time because vessels naturally lose some of their flexibility. This less movement can make it harder for blood to flow and raise blood pressure.

Plaque Buildup: Years of being around risk factors like high cholesterol can cause plaque to slowly build up in the airways.

Weakened Heart Muscle: As people get older, their heart muscles can get weaker, making them less able to pump blood.

Even though chronological age can't be changed, knowing that this increases the chance means that other risk factors can be watched more closely and dealt with earlier.

The Heart of Life: How Genes Affect Heart Health

Your genetics can affect how likely you are to get heart disease. Some genes can affect how much cholesterol is in the blood, how well blood pressure is controlled, and how well the heart muscle works. Your risk of getting heart disease is greatly raised if someone close to you, like a parent or child, has had it before.

Genes are not, however, fate. Adopting a heart-healthy lifestyle can greatly lower your risk of getting heart disease, even if you are genetically more likely to get it.

Out of Your Hands: Your Family History and How It Affects You

Heart disease is more likely to happen if you have a family background of it. You are more likely to get heart disease if a parent, sibling, or kid has it, especially if they are young. A person's genes and things in their environment, like their diet and lifestyle, are likely to work together to make this chance higher.

When you know your family background, you have the power to act. Talk to your doctor about any health problems that run in your family and get checked for things like high blood pressure and cholesterol. Finding and treating heart problems early on are very important if you have a family history of heart problems.

Living with Risk Factors You Can't Control: Prevention Methods

You can't change your age, your genes, or your family background, but there are things you can do to take charge of your heart health:

Early detection and monitoring: It's important to see your doctor regularly for checkups. This includes checking your blood pressure and cholesterol levels and talking to your doctor about any signs that worry you.

Changes to your lifestyle: Pay attention to risk factors that you can control. Maintain a healthy weight, do regular physical exercise, eat a heart-healthy diet, deal with stress, and don't smoke. Even if there are things you can't change, these healthy habits can still lower your chance by a lot.

Medicines: If you have other health problems, like high blood pressure or cholesterol, taking medications as prescribed by your doctor can greatly lower your risk of issues from heart disease.

Open Communication with Your Doctor: Tell your doctor everything you know about your family background and any worries you have. Talking to your doctor about your risk factors for heart disease lets you take a personalized approach to preventing it.

Remember that you can have a big impact on your heart health even if you can't change some of the risk factors that put you at risk. You can do this by finding problems early, taking action to fix them, and committing to a healthy lifestyle.

In conclusion

Age, DNA, and a history of heart disease are all risk factors for heart disease that you can't change, but they don't have to decide your future. Knowing about these things and taking action can give you the power to take good care of your heart health. Heart disease and its problems are much less likely to happen if you get them caught early, live a healthy lifestyle, and maybe even take medicine. The best way to live a long and healthy life is to take care of your health, no

matter what.

Chapter 6

Risk Factors That Can Be Changed

Lifestyle Choices You Can Make

Heart disease is the top cause of death in the world, but it's not a given. Luckily, many of the things that put us at risk for heart disease can be changed by the choices we make every day. This chapter gives you power by talking about the changeable risk factors, or things in your life that you can change to lower your risk of heart disease and improve your overall cardiovascular health.

Fueling Your Heart for Success: What You Eat

A healthy food is the most important part of living a heart-healthy life. What you eat can affect your heart health in these ways:

Bad Fats: Saturated and trans fats, which are found in processed meats, fried foods, and some baked goods, should be avoided. These fats make plaque build up in the airways.

When it comes to cholesterol, red meat, egg yolks, and organ foods are all good sources. Pick lean protein sources like beans, fish, and chicken.

Salt: Eating too much salt can raise blood pressure, which is a major risk factor for heart disease. Choose low-sodium foods instead of processed foods and table salt that has been added.

Added sugars: Sugary drinks and processed foods make you gain weight and inflame your body, which are both bad for your heart. Instead of extra sugars, choose natural sweeteners like fruits.

Eat lots of fruits, vegetables, and whole grains. They are full of vitamins, minerals, and fiber, all of which are good for your heart. Eat more veggies, fruits, and whole grains like quinoa, brown rice, and whole-wheat bread.

A heart-healthy diet is low in unhealthy fats, salt, and added sugars and high in fruits, veggies, whole grains, and lean protein. This will greatly lower your risk of getting heart disease.

Move Your Body: The Power of Exercise

Getting enough exercise is one of the best ways to fight heart disease. This is how daily exercise is good for your heart:

Strengthens the Heart Muscle: When you work out regularly, your heart muscle gets stronger, which lets it pump blood better with each beat.

Improving blood flow: Being active helps your body's blood move well, bringing oxygen and nutrients to your heart and other organs.

Lowers Blood Pressure: Working out helps keep your blood pressure in check, which is good for your heart and vessels.

Controls Weight: Being active regularly can help you keep a healthy weight, which is good for your heart.

Boosts HDL Cholesterol: Working out can raise your HDL ("good") cholesterol levels, which helps get rid of LDL ("bad") cholesterol from your arteries.

Aim for 150 minutes of aerobic exercise at a low level or 75 minutes of aerobic exercise at a high level every week. At least twice a week, you should do strength training routines that work all of your major muscle groups.

Getting the Right Balance: Heart Health and Weight Loss

Being overweight is a major risk factor for heart disease. Why it's important to keep a good weight:

It makes your heart work less hard to pump blood throughout your body. Being overweight makes your heart work harder to do its job.

Lessens Blood Pressure and Cholesterol: Losing weight can lower blood pressure and lower cholesterol, which are both good for heart health.

Lowers Your Risk of Diabetes: Being overweight or obese is a big risk factor for type 2 diabetes, which can raise your risk of heart disease even more.

Having a balanced diet and doing regular physical exercise are both important for keeping your weight at a healthy level.

Giving up smoking is good for your heart

Smoking is one of the main things that can be done to avoid getting heart disease. It's bad for your heart in these ways:

Hurts Blood Vessels: Smoking hurts the walls of your arteries, which makes them more likely to get plaque buildup.

Blood Pressure Goes Up: Smoking makes your blood vessels narrow and your blood pressure go up, which puts more stress on your heart.

Less Oxygen: When you smoke, your blood doesn't carry as much oxygen, which means your heart and other systems don't get enough oxygen.

One of the most important things you can do to improve your heart health is to stop smoking. Talk to your doctor about ways to get help and tools to help you stop smoking for good.

Less stress, more life: how to deal with stress for a healthy heart

Stress that lasts for a long time can hurt your heart. Here are some ways that worry can hurt your heart:

Blood Pressure Goes Up: Hormones that cause stress, like cortisol, can temporarily raise blood pressure. Heart disease is more likely to happen if you have high blood pressure all the time.

Risk of Unhealthy Habits: Stress can make people overeat, smoke, or use other unhealthy ways to deal with their problems, all of which raise the risk of heart disease.

There are, thankfully, healthy ways to deal with worry and keep your heart healthy:

Techniques for Relaxation: Yoga, meditation, and deep breathing are some practices that can help calm the body and mind, which can lower stress.

Support from friends and family: Having strong friendships can help you deal with stress. Spend time with family and friends, and make a group of people who can help you.

Healthy Sleep Habits: Try to get between 7 and 8 hours of good sleep every night. Getting enough sleep helps your mind and body recharge, which makes it easier to deal with worry.

Time Management: Figure out how to organize your time and set priorities. Being too busy can make you feel stressed.

Get Professional Help: If worry is getting to be too much for you to handle on your own, don't be afraid to get help from a therapist or counselor.

It is possible to greatly lower your risk of heart disease and improve your general health by learning how to deal with stress.

Giving yourself the tools you need for a heart-healthy lifestyle

The good news is that you can make a big difference in how healthy your heart is. By making heart-healthy choices about your diet, amount of physical activity, weight, quitting smoking, and dealing with stress, you can greatly lower your chances of getting heart disease.

Don't forget that little changes can have big effects. Start by making small changes to your practice that you can keep up. Build on these small wins over time, and you'll be well on your way to living a heart-healthy life.

You can live a long and healthy life if you take care of your health and make smart choices. This chapter has given you the information and tools you need to make smart choices that will keep your heart healthy in the future. The following chapters will go into more detail about the tests used to find heart disease, the different types of heart problems that can be treated, and how important it is to live a healthy life in order to control heart disease.

Part 4

Taking Charge

Strategies for Stopping Heart Disease

Chapter 7
How to Eat Well for Your Heart
Food as Medicine

An old proverb says, "You are what you eat." This is especially true when it comes to heart health. A heart-healthy diet full of certain nutrients and whole foods can lower your risk of heart disease by a lot and help your heart stay healthy. This chapter will talk about the idea of food as medicine, the specific parts of a healthy diet that are good for your heart, and how to make a heart-healthy eating plan.

A powerful way to improve heart health is to use food as medicine.

The food you eat is like a treasure chest full of heart-healthy tools. The right kinds of food can help with

Lower your blood pressure

Bring down cholesterol levels

Lower the redness

For good blood flow,

Stay at a good weight.

When you eat these heart-healthy foods, you're not just getting food to stay alive; you're also strengthening your heart and making it healthier.

Important Foods for a Heart-Healthy Heart

Now let's talk about the foods that are most important for a heart-healthy diet:

Foods that are bright and colorful: these are full of vitamins, minerals, fiber, and antioxidants. Aim for a rainbow on your plate by eating different kinds of fruits and veggies all day long.

A plate of brightly colored fruits and veggies

Whole Grains: Whole grains, like brown rice, quinoa, and whole-wheat bread, are a great way to get fiber, complex carbs, and minerals and vitamins your body needs. Whole grains give you long-lasting energy and help keep your blood sugar levels in check, which lowers your risk of diabetes, which in turn lowers your risk of heart disease.

Lean Protein: Fish, chicken, beans, and lentils are all good sources of lean protein. Omega-3 fatty acids are good for your heart and can be found in large amounts in fish, especially heavy fish like salmon, tuna, and mackerel. Omega-3s lower inflammation, make blood move better, and may even help lower triglycerides and blood pressure.

Healthy Fats: Not all fats are the same. Avocados, nuts, seeds, and olive oil are all good sources of healthy fats that are good for your heart. These fats help cut down on "bad" LDL cholesterol and raise "good" HDL cholesterol.

In fruits, veggies, whole grains, and legumes, you can find fiber. Fiber is very important for heart health. Fiber keeps your gut system healthy and helps keep your blood sugar and cholesterol levels in check.

Building a Heart-Healthy Plate: Useful Hints

Let's add these heart-healthy heroes to a tasty and well-balanced diet now that you know who they are:

Half of Your Plate Should Be Fruits and veggies: At every meal, fill half of your plate with different colored fruits and veggies. This will make sure you get enough fiber, vitamins, and minerals.

You should eat whole grains instead of sweetened grains. Instead of white bread and rice, you should eat brown rice, quinoa, and whole-wheat bread. Whole grains give you energy that lasts and make you feel full for longer.

Choose lean types of protein, such as grilled chicken, fish, beans, and lentils. Cut back on red meat, processed foods, and bad sources of saturated fat.

Accept Healthy Fats: Eat foods like olive oil, nuts, seeds, avocados, and avocados that are high in healthy fats. You can drizzle and cook with olive oil, and nuts and seeds are a great snack.

Limit Added Sugars and salt: Watch out for processed foods that have a lot of added sugars and salt. Carefully read food labels and pick choices that have less of these bad ingredients.

Cook More at Home: When you cook at home, you can choose what goes into your food and how much you eat. Try out some healthy meals and find new ones that you like.

Don't Forget to Watch Your Portions: Even healthy foods can be bad for you if you eat too much of them. Mindful eating means paying attention to when your body tells you it's hungry or full.

An example of a heart-healthy meal plan

You can start your heart-healthy journey with this sample meal plan:

I ate oatmeal with nuts and berries for breakfast and Greek yogurt with fruit and granola for lunch.

Served for lunch, a salad with grilled chicken or fish and a whole-wheat wrap with fruit and lean protein.

Tonight for dinner, I'm having salmon with roasted veggies and lentil soup with white bread.

Fruits, veggies with hummus, nuts, and seeds are good snacks.

Don't forget that this is only a taste. Feel free to change it to suit your tastes and food needs.

Adopt a lifestyle that is good for your heart

A heart-healthy diet isn't just about following rules; it's about eating in a way that is good for your body and tastes great. Fruits, veggies, whole grains, lean protein, and healthy fats are all heart-healthy foods that you can add to your meals. This will help you live a tasty and heart-healthy life.

Always being the same is important. Over time, small changes that can be kept up will have big effects. Don't let rare mistakes get you down; see them as chances to learn and get back on track right away.

Eating in a way that is good for your heart is like putting money into your future. A better body, a healthier heart, and a full life are the benefits. We'll talk about the testing tools used to find heart disease in the next chapter, which will

give you the knowledge to take charge of your heart health.

Chapter 8
Move Your Body
How Exercise Can Help Your Heart

The muscle in your heart works best when you work it out regularly, just like any other muscle. We'll talk more about how powerful exercise is for heart health in this chapter. We'll talk about the different kinds of exercise that are good for your heart, give you ideas for how to make movement a part of your daily life, and encourage you to get moving to become healthier and happy.

A natural way to keep your heart healthy is to work out. Being active is an important part of living a heart-healthy life. This is how daily exercise is good for your heart:

Stronger Heart Muscle: Working out makes your heart muscle stronger and more efficient, which means that each beat it makes, it pumps blood more efficiently. This makes your heart work less hard and improves blood flow all over your body.

Improves Blood Flow: Being active helps your blood flow well, which brings oxygen and nutrients to your heart and other important systems. This blood is full of oxygen, which keeps your heart working well.

Lowers Blood Pressure: Working out regularly can help keep your blood pressure in check, which is good for your heart and vessels.

Controls Weight: Working out helps you keep a healthy weight, which is important for making your heart less stressed. When you are overweight, your heart has to work harder to get blood to all parts of your body.

Increases HDL Cholesterol: Working out can raise your HDL ("good") cholesterol levels, which helps get rid of LDL ("bad") cholesterol from your arteries. This lowers the risk of heart disease and plaque buildup.

Reduces Inflammation: Being active regularly can help fight chronic inflammation, which is a major risk factor for heart disease.

There's no doubt that exercise is good for your heart. One of the best ways to avoid heart disease and improve your overall health is to make regular physical exercise a part of your life.

Learning How to Get Fit: Different Exercises

There isn't a single way to exercise that works for everyone. The important thing is to find things you enjoy doing and can make a regular part of your life. Here are some great ways to workout that are good for your heart:

Cardio, which is another name for physical exercise, raises your heart rate and keeps it there for a long time. Some examples are walking quickly, running, swimming, riding a bike, and dancing. Aim for 150 minutes of aerobic exercise at a low level or 75 minutes of aerobic exercise at a high level every week.

Strength training: Not only does it make you look better, but it's also good for your heart. At least twice a week, you should do strength training routines that work all of your major muscle groups. You can work out with resistance bands, free weights, or your own body.

Low-Impact Activities: Walking, swimming, and yoga are all great low-impact workouts that you can do if you have limitations or are just starting out. Even though they are easy on the joints, these exercises are still good for your heart. Finding things you enjoy and can do for a long time is the most important thing.

Making working out a habit: ways to get moving every day

A lot of people find it hard to start an exercise routine, but even small changes can become big ones. Here are some ways to make moving a part of your daily life:

Start small and build up slowly: Don't try to change everything about your habit all at once. Start with short bursts of movement, like 10-minute walks. As your fitness level rises, slowly add more time and intensity to your workouts.

Find an Exercise Buddy: Working out with a family member or friend can keep you motivated and hold you accountable. You can hold each other responsible and enjoy working out more.

Make it Fun: Pick things you really love doing. Try something new, like dancing, hiking, or team sports. You're more likely to keep up with exercise if it's fun.

Do something active every day. For example, instead of taking the lift, park farther away and walk, or stretch or do bodyweight exercises during commercial breaks while watching TV. Every little bit of moving counts!

Track Your Progress: Seeing how far you've come can really push you to do better. You can use a fitness watch, write down your workouts, or just pay attention to how you feel as you get fitter.

Always being the same is important. Aim to work out at a reasonable level for at least 30 minutes most days of the week. Little bursts of exercise throughout the day can make a big difference in the health of your heart.

Outside the Gym: Everyday Activities to Make Your Life More Active

You don't have to go to the gym to work out. Here are some ways to make moving a part of your everyday:

During breaks at work, get up and move around every half hour to an hour. Stretch, go up and down the stairs a few times, or walk around the office.

Do Household Chores with Vigor: Do work around the house like cleaning, gardening, or yard work as short workouts. Play some music and move around some!

Whenever you can, take the stairs instead of the elevator. This is an easy but effective way to get more exercise during the day.

Fitness Fun for the Whole Family: Take your family on active trips like hikes, biking, swimming, or playing active games in the park.

Adding these everyday things to your routine will help you move around more and keep your heart healthy.

Moving around will make your heart healthier.

Regular exercise is one of the best ways to keep your heart healthy. By moving, you make your heart muscle stronger, improve blood flow, keep your weight in check, and lower your risk of getting heart disease. You don't have to spend hours at the gym to get rid of those bad habits. You can slowly get fitter by doing things you enjoy and making moving a part of your daily life.

Making small changes to your daily routine will help your heart stay healthy. We'll talk about the diagnostic tools used to find heart problems in the next chapter. With this information, you can take charge of your heart health and spot any problems before they get worse.

Part 5

Optimizing Your Health

Lifestyle Habits for Prevention

Chapter 9
How to Control Your Weight
Finding a Healthy Balance

Keeping your weight at a good level is very important for heart health. Having too much weight puts stress on your heart and makes you more likely to get heart disease. This chapter talks about how managing your weight can help your heart health, looks at good ways to lose weight, and stresses how important it is to find a balance that you can keep up for long-term success.

Why your heart cares about your weight (The Weighty Connection)

Heart disease is more likely to happen if you are overweight, especially around your middle. This is how being overweight can hurt your heart health:

Stress on the Heart: Being overweight makes your heart work harder to pump blood around your body, which can damage its performance.

High Blood Pressure: Being overweight or obese makes you more likely to have high blood pressure, which can damage your arteries and make you more likely to have a heart attack or stroke.

Blood Sugar Control Problems: Being overweight can make insulin resistance worse, which can lead to type 2 diabetes and raise your chance of heart disease even more.

Bad Cholesterol Levels: Being overweight can cause LDL ("bad") cholesterol levels to rise and HDL ("good") cholesterol levels to fall, which is not a healthy mix.

Chronic Inflammation: Being overweight can cause inflammation all over the body, which can hurt blood vessels and raise the risk of heart disease.

Keeping a healthy weight is important for lowering your chance of heart disease and improving your heart health in general.

How to Find Your Healthy Weight

The first step to managing your weight well is to know your healthy weight range. People often use these two tools to find a good weight range:

Body Mass Index (BMI): Your height and weight are used to figure out your BMI, which tells you how much body fat you have. But it's important to remember that BMI doesn't tell the difference between muscle mass and fat mass, and it might not be right for everyone, especially athletes or people who have a lot of muscle mass.

Waist Circumference: Your waist circumference can tell you a lot about your belly fat, which is very bad for your heart health. Men whose waists are bigger than 40 inches (102 cm) and women whose waists are bigger than 35 inches (88 cm) are thought to be more likely to get heart disease.

Talk to your doctor about what weight range is good for you, taking into account your body type and health history.

Sustainable Ways to Lose Weight: Losing Weight for a Healthier Heart

If you want to lose weight, you should focus on long-term plans that help you form good habits. These are some important rules:

Food and Exercise: A healthy way to lose weight is to eat a balanced diet and do regular physical exercise. A healthy diet should include lots of fruits, veggies, whole grains, and lean protein. You should also try to eat less processed foods, unhealthy fats, and added sugars. As part of your usual exercise, do both cardio and strength training.

Measure Your Portion Sizes: Watch how much you eat. Use smaller plates and don't snack without thinking.

Slow down and enjoy your food with mindful eating. Don't eat too much; just until you're full.

Discover Activities You Enjoy: Do physical activities you enjoy, and you'll be more likely to keep up with them over time.

Set Realistic Goals: If you want to lose weight, set small goals that you can reach. Don't let failures get you down; instead, celebrate your wins along the way.

Don't forget that losing weight is a process, not a goal. Make it a point to form healthy habits that you will keep up forever.

Creating Habits That Will Last for Long-Term Success

Here's how to make habits that will last and help you keep your weight down and keep your heart healthy:

Plan Your Meals: Making plans for your meals and snacks ahead of time can help you stay on track with healthy choices and resist the urge to eat something unhealthy.

Cook More at Home: When you cook at home, you can choose what goes into your food and how much you eat.

Read Food Labels: Be aware of what you're eating by reading food labels and picking foods that are lower in salt, added sugars, and unhealthy fats.

Stay Hydrated: Lots of water can help you feel full and cut down on the number of calories you eat.

Take care of your stress: long-term worry can make you eat poorly. To deal with stress in a healthy way, do things like exercise, learn how to relax, or spend time with people you care about.

Get Enough Sleep: Try to get 7-8 hours of good sleep every night. Getting enough sleep helps keep hormones in check, which affects hunger and weight control.

Do Not Deprive Yourself: Give yourself treats every once in a while, but not too many. Feeling deprived can make you want to eat too much.

If you follow these tips and make healthy habits a part of your life, you can reach and keep a healthy weight, which will lower your risk of heart disease and improve your general health.

Finding Balance for a Heart and Life That Are Healthy

Keeping your weight in check is very important for heart health. However, it's important to keep things in check. Not just losing weight on the scale is important; you should also focus on making habits that will last and improve your health in the long run. Enjoy your growth, live a healthy life, and don't let setbacks get you down. Getting your weight down is always good for your heart.

We'll learn more about the tools and tests used to find heart problems in the next chapter, which is all about diagnostics. For treatment and care to work, early detection is key. This gives you the power to take charge of your heart health.

Chapter 10

Seeing the Enemy

Heart Disease Diagnostic Tools

Even though heart illness is complicated, it can be found. This chapter will talk about the different testing tools and tests that are used to find heart disease and possible risk factors. For treatment and care to work, early detection is key. This gives you the power to take charge of your heart health.

Why early detection is important

Finding heart disease early lets you get help and care right away, which greatly increases your chances of living a healthy and happy life. This is why early discovery is so important:

Early intervention: If heart disease is found early, treatment can start right away, which may help avoid complications and improve long-term results.

Management of risk factors: If you and your doctor find the disease early, you can take care of underlying risk factors like high blood pressure, high cholesterol, or diabetes, which stops the disease from getting worse.

Changing your lifestyle: An early diagnosis can wake you up and inspire you to make healthy changes to your food, exercise, and how you deal with stress, all of which can greatly improve your heart health.

If you find heart disease early, you can take charge of your health and avoid problems in the future.

Diagnostic Tools That Your Doctor Can Use

Here are some of the tools and tests that your doctor might use to find out if you have heart disease:

Medical History and Physical Exam: Your doctor will talk to you about your present symptoms, medical history, and any family history of heart disease. During a physical checkup, your blood pressure, heart rate, and heart sound may be checked for any problems.

Blood Tests: Cholesterol, blood sugar, and inflammation markers can all be found in blood tests, and they can all show if someone is at risk for heart disease.

Electrocardiogram (ECG): An ECG is a quick and easy test that checks how your heart is working electrically. It can find heart rate problems or damage to the heart muscle.

Echocardiogram (Echo): Ultrasound waves are used in an echo to make pictures of your heart. This test can find out how big your heart valves and chambers are and how well they work.

Chest X-ray: A chest X-ray can give a general picture of your heart and lungs. It may show signs of an enlarged heart or fluid buildup in the lungs.

Stress Test: During a stress test, your heart rate, blood pressure, and electrical activity are tracked while you move or take medicine that makes you feel like you're exercising. This test can tell you how well your heart handles stress.

In cardiac catheterization, a thin tube is put into an artery or vein and guided to the heart. This is a more invasive process. It gives you a clear picture of your coronary arteries and can be used for treatments like angioplasty or stent placement.

Based on your symptoms and risk factors, your doctor will tell you what tests to get.

What You Know Can Make a Difference in Your Heart Health

One of the best ways to fight heart disease is to find it early. This information gives you power in these ways:

Proactive approach: If you find heart problems early, you can take charge of your health. You can make changes to your lifestyle and work with your doctor to make a specific treatment plan. This will lower your risk of complications.

Peace of mind: Being aware of your heart health can give you peace of mind. If no problems are found, you can focus on living a healthy life to keep problems from happening in the future.

Empowerment: Finding a problem early gives you the power to be involved in your own health care. You can ask questions, learn about your care options, and make health-related choices that are best for you.

Don't wait until you start to feel sick. Get regular checkups with your doctor and talk about the things that put you at risk for heart disease.

Getting to the bottom of the enemy for a healthier you

Finding heart problems early is very important for effective treatment and management. Your doctor can get a full picture of your heart health with the testing tools they have access to. You can take care of your heart health and live a long, healthy life if you know what puts you at risk and work with your doctor.

In the next part, we'll talk about different ways to treat heart conditions, giving you more information about what you can do.

Part 6

Beyond Lifestyle

Medical Interventions for Heart Disease

Chapter 11
Medicines For Heart Health
Learning About Your Choices

Heart disease is a strong enemy, but it can be defeated. There are a lot of medicines that can help people with different heart diseases control their symptoms and keep complications from happening. This chapter tells you about the different types of heart medicines and how they can help your heart stay healthy.

A targeted approach: medicines for certain health problems

Heart disease includes a wide range of conditions, and medicines are made to treat particular problems:

High Blood Pressure: ACE inhibitors, angiotensin II receptor blockers (ARBs), calcium channel blockers, diuretics, and beta-blockers are some of the medicines that are often used to lower blood pressure and make the heart work less hard.

High Cholesterol: Statins are the most common type of medicine used to lower cholesterol. The way they work is by stopping the liver from making LDL ("bad") cholesterol.

Coronary Artery Disease: Aspirin and clopidogrel are examples of antiplatelet drugs that help keep blood from clotting, which can lead to heart attacks or strokes. For better blood flow to the heart, nitrates are used to loosen up blood arteries.

Heart Failure: ACE inhibitors, ARBs, and beta-blockers help the heart pump more efficiently by reducing the amount of work it has to do. Diuretics help the body get rid of extra fluid.

Arrhythmias are irregular heartbeats. Beta-blockers, calcium channel blockers, and antiarrhythmic drugs can help keep the heart rhythm normal and avoid problems.

It's important to remember that this isn't a full list, and that you should only take medicines as directed by a doctor.

Learning About the Pros and Cons of Medicine

Taking medicines for heart health can make your life a lot better. If you want to know more about their pros and cons, read on:

Benefits: Medicines can lower cholesterol, blood pressure, and heart rate, improve blood flow, stop blood clots, and ease symptoms like chest pain and shortness of breath.

Side Effects: Heart medicines can have side effects, just like any other medicine. These can be different for each person and each drug. Tiredness, dizziness, headaches, and stomachaches are some of the most common side effects. It's important to talk to your doctor about possible side effects and share any that bother you.

Being honest with your doctor is important for dealing with side effects and getting the most out of your medications.

Taking medication and living a healthy life

Medicines work very well, but they're not a magic bullet. For them to work best and improve general heart health, you need to live a healthy life:

Diet: Eat a heart-healthy diet full of fruits, veggies, whole grains, and lean protein, and cut back on bad fats, added sugars, and sodium.

Exercise: Do regular physical exercise based on what your doctor tells you.

Managing your weight: Keeping your weight at a healthy level makes your heart work better.

Stress Management: Dealing with stress in a healthy way is important because long-term worry can make heart problems worse.

Quitting smoking: If you smoke, this is the most important thing you can do for your heart health.

Taking your medicine and living a healthy life together can greatly lower your risk of heart problems and help you live a long and happy life.

Working with your doctor to get the best heart health

Medication is an important part of controlling heart disease, but it works best when used along with a healthy lifestyle.

Talk to your doctor about any worries or questions you have about the medicines you take. To make a treatment plan that improves your heart health and general well-being, you need to be able to talk to your doctor and work together.

The last part of this book will talk about the power of prevention and stress how important it is to make healthy choices every day to protect your heart for years to come.

Chapter 12

When Lifestyle Changes Aren't Enough

Procedures And Interventions

A heart-healthy way of life is the most important thing you can do to avoid and control heart disease. But sometimes, making changes to your habits may not be enough. This chapter talks about the different methods and interventions that are used to treat heart problems and make heart health better.

A Range of Interventions Besides Medication

If medicines and changes to your lifestyle aren't enough to control your heart disease, your doctor may suggest slightly invasive procedures or surgeries. Here is a list of some usual interventions:

coronary angioplasty and stent placement: This method is used to clear out coronary vessels that are blocked. A thin tube with a balloon on the end is put into the artery and filled to make the blockage bigger. To keep the artery open, a stent, which is a small metal tube, may be put in place.

Coronary Artery Bypass Grafting (CABG): In CABG, a healthy blood line from another part of the body is grafted to go around a blocked coronary artery. This makes the heart muscle get more blood.

Repair or Replacement of a Valve: If a heart valve is broken or not working right, it may need to be fixed or changed with a fake valve. This might help the heart pump blood better.

If you have an arrhythmia (irregular heartbeat), an implantable cardioverter-defibrillator (ICD) or a pacemaker can help keep your heart beating normally. A pacemaker sends electrical signals to the heart to keep it beating at a regular rate. An ICD, on the other hand, can correct a heartbeat that is too fast and could be dangerous.

LVAD stands for Left Ventricular Assist Device. An LVAD is an artificial pump that is put into the chest to help a heart that isn't working as well pump blood around the body. It's often used as a step toward a heart transplant or for people who can't get a transplant.

Heart Transplant: If you have serious heart failure, you might need a heart transplant. A healthy donor heart is put in place of the sick heart during this surgery.

The treatment your doctor suggests will depend on what kind of heart problem you have and how bad it is.

Taking into account the pros and cons of interventions

Surgery and medical treatments can save lives, but they can also be dangerous. Take a look at these things:

Benefits: Interventions and procedures can improve blood flow to the heart, ease chest pain and shortness of breath, and make life better in general.

Risks: There are some risks that come with every treatment, like bleeding, getting an infection, or having problems during surgery. It's important to talk to your doctor in detail about these risks before going ahead with the plan.

For your specific case, your doctor will help you weigh the possible pros and cons of any action to find the best way to proceed.

Recovery and Getting Better After Surgery

A good recovery process is very important after a heart procedure or surgery. To do this, you might:

Hospitalization: For tracking and care during the first few days after surgery, you may need to stay in the hospital.

Cardiac Rehabilitation: After a heart attack or stroke, cardiac rehabilitation is a personalized program that helps you get stronger and improve your heart health. It usually includes learning how to exercise, getting information on how to deal with heart disease, and getting mental support.

Medication: After surgery, you may need to keep taking medications to control your heart disease.

Changes to your lifestyle: After surgery, living a healthy life is even more important to avoid problems in the future. This includes eating well, working out daily, dealing with stress, and giving up smoking.

For a good result after a cardiac procedure, you must follow your doctor's recovery plan and make the changes they suggest to your lifestyle.

In conclusion: A Team Approach to the Best Heart Health

Taking care of complicated heart problems often needs a team effort. Your doctor and other medical professionals, such as nurses, cardiac rehabilitation experts, and therapists, will work together to make a personalized treatment plan for you. This plan may include changes to your lifestyle, medications, and maybe even procedures or interventions. This is the best thing that can happen for your heart health: you work together.

The last chapter of this book will be a concluding lesson that stresses how important it is to live a heart-healthy life for life.

Part 7

Living Well with Heart Disease

A Guide to Long-Term Management

Chapter 13

You Will Be Committed To Heart Health For The Rest Of Your Life

Even though heart disease is strong, you are not helpless. We've talked a lot about how important a healthy living is for preventing and treating heart disease in this book. This last chapter is a call to action that will give you the tools to make decisions that will protect your heart for a lifetime.

The Power of Not Doing It: The Power of One Ounce...

It's true that "an ounce of prevention is worth a pound of cure" when it comes to heart health. Living a heart-healthy life can make it much less likely that you will get heart disease in the first place. This is how prevention gives you power:

Less danger: Living a healthy life can make it much less likely that you will get heart disease, high blood pressure, high cholesterol, and other problems.

Better quality of life: Eating healthy foods, working out regularly, and dealing with stress are all healthy habits that can give you more energy, make you feel better, and improve your general health.

Taking preventative steps for your health puts you in charge and gives you power. You are taking steps to keep your heart healthy and improve your long-term health.

Prevention isn't just about staying away from sickness; it's also about building a strong base for a full and healthy life.

The Three Keys to Prevention: How to Make Your Heart Healthy

A heart-healthy way of life doesn't involve big changes or trendy meals. Making habits that you can keep up for life is what it's all about. The most important things for protection are:

A Good Diet: A healthy diet should include lots of fruits, veggies, whole grains, and lean protein. Cut back on processed foods, unhealthy fats, and extra sugars.

Strive to work out at least 150 minutes a week at a low level of intensity or 75 minutes a week at a high level of intensity. Discover things you enjoy doing and slowly get more active.

Managing your weight: Keeping your weight at a healthy level makes your heart work better. Focus on eating well and working out to keep the weight off for good.

Managing your stress: Long-term worry can hurt your heart health. To deal with stress in a healthy way, try yoga, relaxation methods, or spending time in nature.

How to Stop Smoking: Smoking increases your chance of heart disease. The best thing you can do for your heart health is to stop smoking.

Keep getting checkups: See your doctor regularly for checkups to keep an eye on your cholesterol, blood pressure, and heart health in general. Early identification is very important for treatment to work and to avoid problems.

There is a good chance that you will avoid heart disease and live a long, healthy life if you follow these prevention steps every day.

Creating a Green Way of Life: Little Changes That Make a Big Difference

Making small, steady changes that you can keep up over time is the key to living a heart-healthy life. Here are some ideas:

Start out small: Don't try to change everything about your life all at once. Start with small goals that you can reach, like eating more veggies or going for a 10-minute walk every day.

Find things you like to do: Eating well and working out shouldn't feel like a burden. Pick things you enjoy doing so you're more likely to keep up with them.

Change things slowly: Over time, slowly make small changes to your diet and gradually raise the intensity and length of your workouts.

Honor your accomplishments: No matter how small your growth is, feel good about it and celebrate it. This will help you keep going on your journey.

Don't give up when things go wrong: Setbacks happen to everyone. You shouldn't give up; instead, get back on track and keep going.

Always being the same is important. You can make small changes to your living that will help your heart health for years to come by making these changes.

In conclusion: Your heart is an amazing engine that will take you through life.

Remember that your heart is an amazing machine that pumps blood all over your body, giving every cell air and nutrients. It's something that keeps your body and mind healthy. We've talked about how complicated heart disease is, how powerful protection is, and how important it is to find and treat heart disease early.

Taking Charge of Your Heart Health: Knowledge Gives You Power

You can take care of your heart health now that you know more about it. You can: Make smart choices about your lifestyle: You now know that what you eat, how much you move, how you deal with stress, and giving up smoking can have a big effect on your heart health.

Take an active role in your health care by: Talk to your doctor about your worries and questions, and work together to make a specific plan for the best heart health.

Push for steps to stop problems: To protect your heart for years to come, make sure you get regular checkups, get screened for risk factors, and put preventative steps at the top of your list.

A promise for life: a heart-healthy future

A heart-healthy lifestyle takes a lifetime to maintain, but the benefits are endless. Putting your heart health first is like investing in a bright future full of energy, health, and the freedom to live life to the fullest.

Don't forget that you're not going through this trip by yourself. Support and encouragement can come from your doctor, other health care workers, and friends and family. Adopt a healthy lifestyle, enjoy your wins, and don't let failures get you down. With hard work and the new information you've learned, you can give yourself the tools you need to live a long, happy life with a strong heart.

Chapter 14

Keeping Your Physical And Mental Health In Good Shape To Live a Fulfilling Life

This chapter shows a change toward a health-focused view that looks at the whole person. The previous chapters were mostly about heart health. This chapter broadens the focus to include the link between physical and mental health, focusing on how both affect living a full life.

The Mind-Body Link: A Dance for Health and Happiness

There are many connections between mental and physical health. What changes one changes the other. This is how they dance together:

Being active makes you feel better: Endorphins are natural chemicals that make you feel good. They fight stress and worry and make you feel good about your health.

The body is affected by long-term stress: Headaches, stomachaches, and a weakened immune system are some of the physical effects of long-term worry.

A healthy diet can help you think more clearly: A healthy diet full of fruits, veggies, and whole grains gives your brain the nutrients it needs to work at its best, which helps you think clearly and concentrate.

Good sleep is good for your health in general: Getting enough sleep is important for both mental and physical recovery. You can handle worry better, concentrate better, and keep your emotional strength when you get enough rest. Taking care of your physical health builds a strong base for your mental health, and the other way around.

Beyond the Body: Important Things for Mental Health

A happy life is more than just being healthy. These are some other things that help to mental health:

Strong social connections: People are social by nature. Having healthy relationships with people you care about gives you a sense of connection, support, and purpose, all of which are good for your mental health.

Mindfulness and Managing Stress: Mindfulness practices, such as yoga or meditation, can help you deal with stress, concentrate better, and find inner peace.

Positive Thinking: Having a positive view on life can improve your mood, strength, and health in general.

Finding Meaning and Purpose: Having a sense of purpose in life, whether it's through work, sports, or volunteering, can make you feel happy and fulfilled.

How to Get Help When You Need It: If you're having problems with your mental health, don't be afraid to get help from a professional. Therapy can help you deal with stress, anxiety, or sadness by giving you tools and plans.

When you take care of your physical and mental health, you build a solid base for a happy and full life.

A set of tools for staying healthy: Easy Ways to Live a Balanced Life

Here are some real-world things you can do to improve your health:

Do physical activities on a regular basis. Pick things you enjoy, like swimming, dancing, brisk walks, or team sports. Aim to work out at least 150 minutes a week at a low level of intensity or 75 minutes a week at a high level of intensity.

Stick to a healthy diet by eating lots of fruits, veggies, whole grains, lean protein, and other unprocessed foods. Cut back on processed foods, unhealthy fats, and extra sugars.

Prioritize Good Sleep: Try to get 7-8 hours of good sleep every night. Set a regular time to go to bed and make a relaxing routine for that time.

Get in touch with family and friends: Take care of your family and friend ties. Plan regular get-togethers with friends and family, have deep talks, and help those you care about.

Use techniques for relaxing: To deal with stress in a healthy way, try yoga, meditation, deep breathing routines, or time spent in nature.

Start a practice of gratitude: Taking the time to enjoy the good things in your life can make you feel better and improve your general health.

Do something new and follow your passions: Your life can feel more purposeful and satisfying if you learn new skills, do hobbies, or help for a cause you care about.

Making these habits a part of your daily life can help you feel good, which is good for your mental and physical health.

In conclusion, your path to a happy life

This book has given you the information and tools you need to put your mental and physical health first. Don't forget that a happy life is a path, not a goal. It will have both good and bad times, challenges and wins. Adopt good habits, enjoy your wins, and don't let setbacks get you down. If you work hard and care about your health, you can build a life full of

energy, meaning, and a strong, healthy heart.